Nouha Farhat

# Cognitive disorders in adult temporal epilepsy

Nouha Farhat

# Cognitive disorders in adult temporal epilepsy

ScienciaScripts

Cover image: www.ingimage.com

This book is a translation from the original published under ISBN 978-620-6-72342-4.

Publisher:
Sciencia Scripts
is a trademark of
Dodo Books Indian Ocean Ltd. and OmniScriptum S.R.L publishing group

120 High Road, East Finchley, London, N2 9ED, United Kingdom
Str. Armeneasca 28/1, office 1, Chisinau MD-2012, Republic of Moldova, Europe
Printed at: see last page
**ISBN: 978-620-8-14102-8**

## CONTENTS

# INTRODUCTION

## INTRODUCTION

Temporal epilepsy (TEE) is a chronic disease characterised by frequent seizures with polymorphic symptoms that are difficult to control with anti-epileptic treatments. Although seizures are the most disabling clinical manifestation, patients with TEE are at risk of associated health problems. Among these co-morbidities, cognitive disorders (CD) are the most common and troublesome. These disorders are now thought to affect 20-50% of patients with ET [1]. The cognitive assessment methods used differ from one study to another. Improved knowledge of neuropsychology, the development of more accurate psychometric tests that are better adapted in terms of function, and the development of assessment scales have all helped to raise awareness of the importance of these cognitive disorders. These have an impact on management (medical and surgical), which led us to take an interest in this subject. In this context, we conducted a prospective study on patients followed in the neurology department of Sfax for diagnosed ET. We tried to detect cognitive complaints during an interview followed by a battery of standardised tests exploring several cognitive domains. We then looked for correlations between these neuropsychological profiles, sociodemographic factors (patient's age, sex, etc.), age of onset of the disease, progression of ET (duration of epilepsy, frequency of seizures, etc.), type and number of treatments, as well as electrical (EEG) and radiological aspects (presence of a lesion, its nature and location (right or left, etc.)).

So, through this work we propose to:

- To study and highlight cognitive impairment in patients with ET.
- Specify the specific cognitive profile of these patients (the areas affected)
- Evaluate the cognitive side effects of treatments to adapt treatment accordingly
- Participate in the process of lateralising and locating the epileptogenic zone

# PATIENTS AND METHODS

# PATIENTS AND METHODS

## 1. Description of the study

This is a cross-sectional study, part of the management of patients with ET at the Habib Bourguiba University Hospital in Sfax over a 12-year period between 1 January 2004 and 30 December 2015. Patients were included prospectively, on the basis of consultation or hospitalisation visits.

We collected epidemiological and clinical data on our patients. We sought to find a correlation between certain factors of the disease (duration of course, time to diagnosis, etc.), the electrical appearance of the EEG, the response to treatment, the aetiology of the epilepsy (location and nature of the lesion) and the presence of CTs.

## 2. Study materials :

### 2.1. Inclusion criteria

We included the following patients in this study:

- Age between 18 and 65
- Follow-up for an ET defined according to the criteria of the International League Against Epilepsy (ILAE)
- Able to take part in a neuropsychological assessment

### 2.2 Exclusion criteria

All patients were excluded from this study:

- suffering from another progressive neurological disease, in particular dementia
- Followed for a psychiatric illness, in particular depression
- Having a brain MRI abnormality other than temporal

## 3. Study methods :

Any patient with ET consulting neurology at the Habib Bourguiba University Hospital between May and November 2022 who met the inclusion criteria and had no exclusion criteria were considered.

### 3.1. Aspects studied :

We drew up a diagnostic form to collect the anamnestic, clinical and para-clinical data for all patients. We specified the following parameters for each patient:

#### 3.1.1. Anamnestic data :

We have specified :

- Epidemiological data (age, gender, level of education)
- Family history of ET
- Personal medical history and current drug treatments
- Age of onset of ET
- How long the disease progresses
- Frequency of CE days
- The nature of the treatment
- The age at which the first TCs appear
- The nature of inaugural CTs and their development

To minimise the risk of interference with our cognitive results, we used a questionnaire to rule out patients with depression: the BECK Abbreviated Questionnaire (BDI), which looks for a possible associated depressive syndrome. A score of 0 to 4 is considered normal.

#### 3.1.2. Neurological examination :

During one of their visits to a neurology consultation or department, we invited patients to take part in this study. Patients who agreed to take part, after giving their informed consent, underwent a clinical examination. All patients underwent a thorough and meticulous neurological examination. Patients were then invited to take part in a specialised neuropsychological assessment based on a battery of standardised tests to determine the presence, nature and severity of CT (the neuropsychological assessment lasted approximately 2 hours).

### 3.1.3. Neuropsychological assessment

We included *thirteen tests* exploring almost all cognitive domains:

Memory :

- ***Verbal episodic memory*** assessed by :
    - *Selective reminiding test (SRT)*, a test for learning and recalling a list of 15 words
    - Grober and Buschke 16-word test (RL / RI-16)
- ***Visual memory*** assessed by :
    - The brief visuo-spatial memory test - revised (BVMT- R)
- ***Short-term memory and working memory***: explored by Empanel test (direct and inverse)

Executive functions: were investigated using 2 tests:

- The "go-no go" test
- TMTA and TMT B tests

Visuospatial functions were examined using 2 tests

- Clock test
- REY figure test

Attention is assessed by

- Bell test

Language is tested by

- Verbal fluency tasks (ISAAC test)

- Denomination (DO80 test)

### 3.1.4. Paraclinical examinations :

#### 3.1.4.1. Electroencephalogram (EEG) :

EEG was performed in all patients followed for ET. We specified the background rhythm and noted whether there were any abnormalities (focal slowing, paroxysmal pathological grapho-elements, etc.).

#### 3.1.4.2. Cerebral MRI :

Brain MRI was routinely performed in all patients with ET

### 3.2. Statistical analysis :

The various data were entered using Microsoft Office Excel 2010 and analysed using SPSS 20 software.

For all statistical tests, the significance level (p) was set at 0.05.

We used :

- Chi 2 test to compare percentages,
- Student's t-test to compare 2 means,
- the bivariate correlation test for comparing 2 quantitative values.

# RESULTS

## RESULTS

We enrolled 32 patients with ET and 30 healthy subjects (controls) matched for age, gender and education.

### 1. Epidemiological data

1.1 ET Group :

1.1.1. Age :

The mean age of our patients was 35 years, ranging from 19 to 92 years. The mean age of onset was 18 years, with extremes ranging from 4 to 60 years. The age distribution showed a peak in frequency between the ages of 35 and 45.

1.1.2. Gender :

In our series, women predominated, with a sex ratio (male/female) of 0.6 (**Figure 1**). There was no statistically significant difference in the age of onset of ET between the 2 sexes (p=0.282).

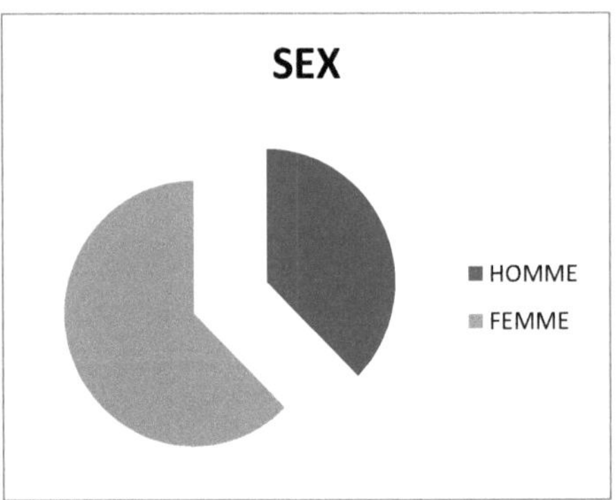


Figure 1: Breakdown of patients by gender.

1.1.3. Educational level :

All our patients had attended school. Eighteen percent had secondary education, while six percent had higher education.

1.1.4. History :

Questioning revealed a family history of epilepsy in 4/32 of the patients, while consanguinity was noted in 5 patients. Febrile seizures occurred in 25% of cases (**Figure 2**).

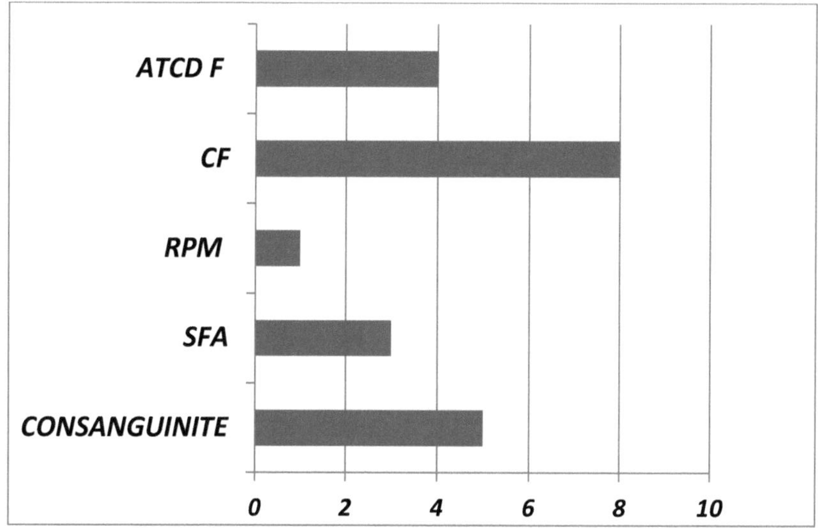


Figure 2: The history of people with epilepsy

1.2 Control groups

This group was matched with the ET group with an average age of our controls of 31.1 years (extremes ranging from 19 to 60 years). In this group, we chose to have more women than men in order to have a sex ratio equal to that of the ET group. All the control subjects had attended school. Of these, the majority (76% of cases) had primary school education. Five subjects had a higher level of education.

2 . Evolution of the disease

2.1. Diffusion of the ZE

The EZ was in the lateral cortex in 8 cases and mesiotemporal in 24 cases.

In ¾ of cases, secondary generalisation of the temporal seizures was observed, and 6.25% had diffusion of the EZ from the temporal cortex to the perisylvian region. The EZ had spread to the frontal cortex in the rest of the epileptics (**Figure 3**).

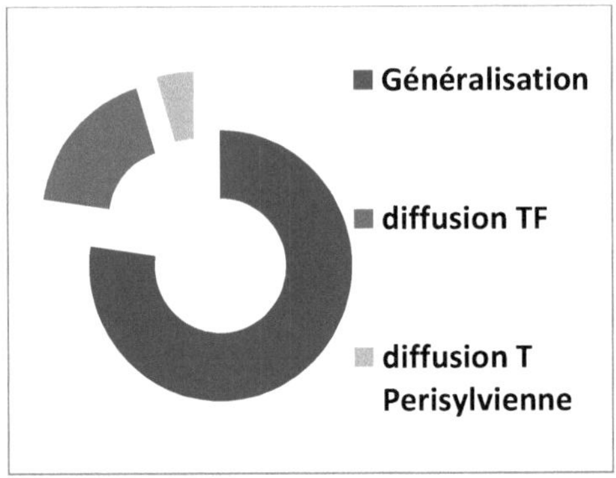


Figure 3: Spread of the epileptogenic zone

2.2. The development time of l'ET

The mean duration of ET was 18.37 years, with extremes ranging from 15 to 32 years.

2.3. Frequency of attacks :

Epilepsy in our series was difficult to control, with an average frequency of one seizure per day.

3. Paraclinical examinations

3.1. THE EEG

The EEG, carried out in all patients, showed diffuse slowing in 6 patients, a focus of slow waves in 10/32 epileptics, and was normal in half the cases.

3.2. Brain MRI

Brain MRI was normal in 6/32 patients and showed abnormalities in the remainder. These anomalies were of various types, such as hippocampal sclerosis in 7 cases (**Figure 6**), vascular anomalies in the same number, cortical dysplasia in 5 epileptics, an expansive process in 4 cases, and temporal cortical dysplasia in 2 cases (**Figure 7**). Radiological signs of left hippocampal atrophy were observed in only one patient (**Figure 5**). The vascular anomalies found in our series were of the cavernoma type in 4/7 patients, while the remaining 3 were ischaemic strokes (2 in the territory of the posterior cerebral artery (Figure 4) and 1 of the anterior choroidal artery). The tumour lesions were also diverse: 2 cases of low-grade glial tumour (Figure no. 8), 1 case of oligodendrocytoma and another of anaplastic ganglioglioma. These abnormalities were right-sided in 12 cases, left-sided in the remaining 13 cases and bilateral in only one case.

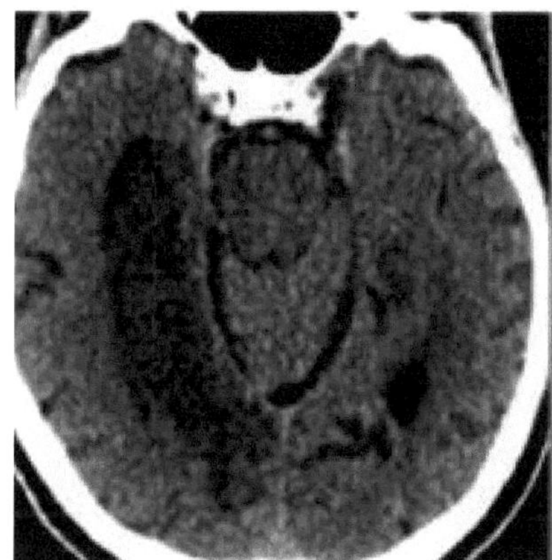

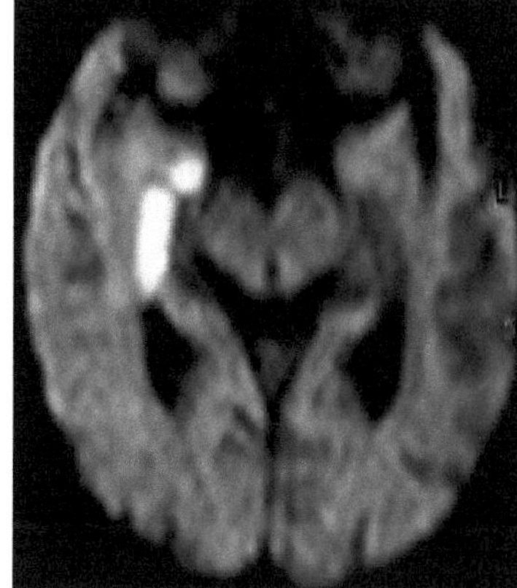

**Figure 4: Axial sections showing right ischaemic stroke in the territory of the right posterior cerebral artery**

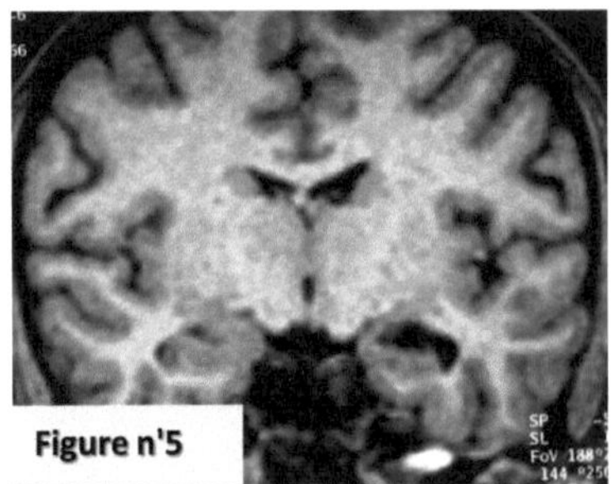


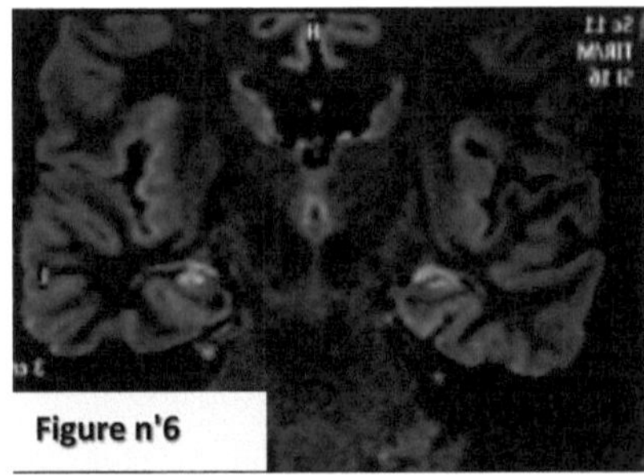


Figure 5: Coronal sections showing left hippocampal atrophy

Figure 6: Coronal sections showing FLAIR hypersignal in the medial part of the 2 temporal lobes in favour of bilateral mesial sclerosis.

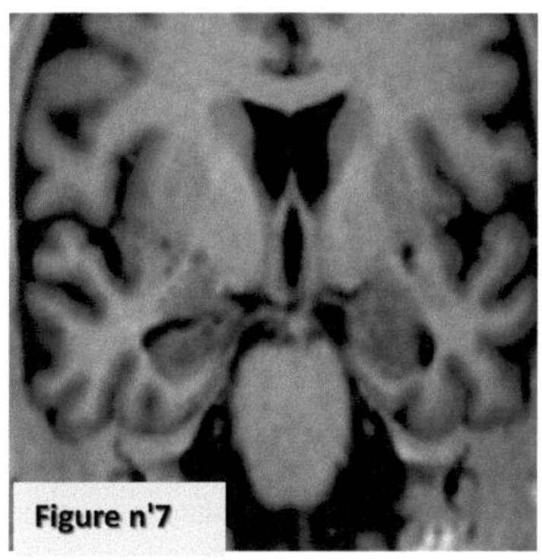


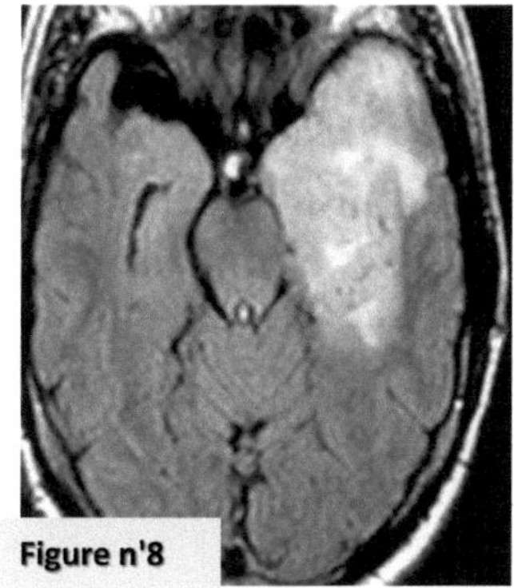


**Figure 7: Coronal inversion-recovery section showing left temporal cortical dysplasia**

**Figure 8: Axial section T2 Flair showing a left temporo-insular infiltrating lesion with T2 hypersignal suggestive of a left low-grade glioma.**

4. Treatment

ET is generally a drug-resistant epilepsy. We found difficulties in balancing the treatment. Only seven patients were on carbamazepine alone. The others were either on dual therapy (12 patients) or polytherapy (13 patients). Carbamazepine was combined with clonazepam in 3 cases and with levetiracetam in 3 others. Sodium valproate was combined with carbamazepine in half the cases. Only 8 of our patients were not on carbamazepine (on a combination of sodium valproate and clonazepam).

5. Cognitive disorders :

5.1. Age and mode of onset of CT

The mean age of onset of cognitive complaints was 28.61 ± 7 years. There was a significantly negative correlation between the age of onset and the severity of cognitive impairment, especially impairment of verbal episodic memory (p=0.001). The first symptoms reported by our patients were memory and concentration problems in 90% of cases. These complaints were inaugural in two patients. The date of onset of these disorders in relation to the diagnosis of the disease varied. The average time to onset in our series was 14 years.

5.2. Cognitive domains affected:

Cognitive disorders affected several domains We observed a slowing down of VTI (100%), attentional disorders (93.57%) and verbal episodic memory (87.5%) as well as visual memory (78.12%). Verbal fluency was impaired in about ¾ of our patients. Working memory was impaired in 53.12%. Executive and visuo-spatial functions were preserved in the majority of cases (**Figure 9**).

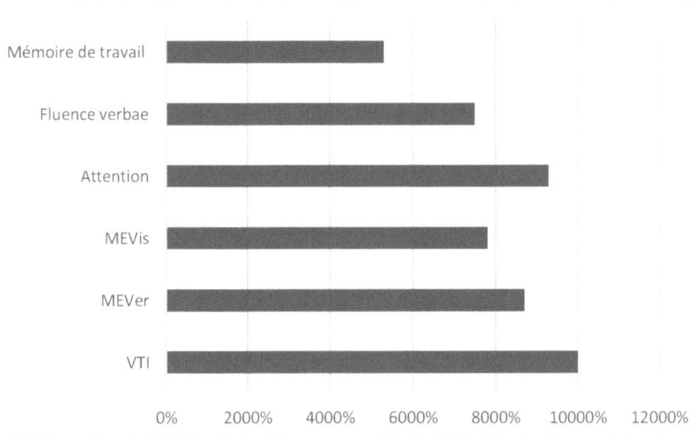


Figure 9: Type of CT in our series

By studying the cognitive domains using various standardised and validated tests, and by comparing the performance of the ET group and the control group, we found that VTI, attention and episodic memory were particularly affected. The abilities of the posterior cognitive domains presented by the visuo-spatial functions were preserved, as were those of the anterior cognitive domains (executive functions).

### 5.2.1. Memory disorders

#### 5.2.1.1. Verbal episodic memory disorders

Impairment of verbal episodic memory was assessed by the 16-word LR/RI test and the 15-word test (SRT). For verbal memory, we found low scores on the 16-word RL/RI test in free recall and total recall compared with the control group, with mean scores of 27.08/48 versus 40.4/48 for free recall (Table I). This test revealed an encoding deficit (the first stage in learning) in 72% of cases compared with control subjects, with a significant difference (p=0.000). Similarly, we concluded that there was a retrieval/restitution deficit in 84.37% of patients assessed by free recall. There was also a statistically significant difference between the control and patient groups in terms of free delayed recall, with scores of 14/16 versus 4/16 (**Table I**).

Table I: RL/RI test scores determined by Grober and Buchke's 16-WORD test.

| SCORE | AND | WITNESSES | P |
|---|---|---|---|
| Immediate recall | 9±4,16 | 15,55 ±0,6 | 0,001 |
| Free recall /48 | 27,08±8 | 40,4± 3,7 | 0,0015 |
| Total recall /48 | 30,76±7,1 | 45,7± 1,8 | 0,002 |
| Free delayed callback/16 | 3.9± 3,8 | 14± 1,8 | 0,042 |
| Indexed delayed callback/16 | 5± 3 | 15,76 ± 0,5 | 0,008 |
| Consolidation score/64 | 31,9±11,4 | 60,8±3 | 0,04 |

Recall capacity assessed by the SRT/15 word test was statistically very impaired (81.5% of cases) (**Table II**).

Table II: Scores for the selective reminding test (SRT)

| SCORE | AND | WITNESSES | P |
|---|---|---|---|
| Immediate recall | 2.38 ±3,791 | 8.61±0,2 | 0,017 |
| Number of words recalled | 68.1±3.9 | 96.7±12,23 | 0,007 |
| Average number of words recalled | 6.1±0.5904 | 12 ±1.9 | 0,006 |
| Learning index/IA | 60±3,7% | 80±12.9% | 0,012 |
| Delayed free recall/15 | 1.37±5,14 | 9.95±2.7 | 0,009 |
| Indexed delayed callback/15 | 1.434 ±0,8 | 15 | 0,000 |

We found that this score was lower in women, but the difference between the two sexes was not significant ($p>0.05$).

5.2.1. 2. Visual episodic memory disorders

Impaired visual episodic memory was assessed by the **BVMT-R** (Brief Visuo-Spatial Memory Test Revised). Compared with normal subjects, 53.12% of patients had low immediate recall scores ($10\leq$ score$\leq20$). As for delayed recall (7min), only 7 patients had scores comparable to controls, i.e. greater than or equal to 8. The difference between the two groups was significant ($p=0.04$). Of the 11 scores that could be obtained using this test, only three were analysed in our study: total recall, delayed recall and recognition. We found that the majority of patients had lower total recall (86%) and delayed recall (76%) scores than the control group, with a significant difference between the two groups (**Table III**).

Table III: BVMT-R test scores

| SCORE | AND | WITNESSES | P |
|---|---|---|---|
| Total recall/ 36 | 23,13±2.8 | 34,47±3,6 | 0,00 |
| Delayed recall/12 | 5,9±3,27 | 11,9±0,3 | 0,04 |
| Recognition | | | |
| Correct answers | 5,44±0,7 | 5,66±0,48 | 0,2 |

| Wrong answers | 0,48±0,7 | 0,33±0,44 | 0,1 |
|---|---|---|---|

5.2.1.3. Short-term memory and working memory disorders :

22 patients had Direct Digit Empan scores comparable to the tans disc 15 controls with the reverse empanel. The extent of these impairments was significant compared with the control group (**Table IV**).

Table IV: EMPAN test scores

| SCORE : | AND | WITNESSES | P |
|---|---|---|---|
| DIRECT/16 | 5 | 10 | 0,02 |
| INVERSE GAP/14 | 4,52 | 9 | 0,01 |

5.2.2. Fluency disorders

Phonological (literal) and semantic verbal fluency were clearly more affected in the patient group than in the control group (**Table V**).

Table V: Scores for the verbal fluency test

| SCORE | AND | WITNESSES | P |
|---|---|---|---|
| Semantic fluency | 15±3,6 | 32,14±4,9 | 0,04 |
| Literal fluency | 7±3,8 | 24±4 | 0,01 |

### 5.2.3. Attention disorders

Compared with control subjects, there was significant impairment of attention, speed and precision in visual search and scanning, as well as attentional capacity in almost all patients (93.57%) with scores<51 (**Table VI**).

The slowdown was evidenced in all patients by a longer total task completion time than the control subjects (> 3min 33sec).

Table VI: Bell test scores (number of correct answers in 120 sec)

| SCORE | AND | WITNESSES | P |
|---|---|---|---|
| Bell (120 sec) | 24,1±12 | 51±7 | 0,02 |

### 5.2.4. Executive disorders

They are mainly investigated by 2 tests: Go no Go and the TMT A and B Test . These tests did not reveal any significant difficulties (**Table VII**).

Table VII: Scores for the Go no Go and TMT tests

| SCORE | AND | WITNESSES | P |
|---|---|---|---|
| **Test GO No GO** | 39,3±1,4 | 40 | 0,3 |
| **TMT A test (score)** | 0.42 | 0.49 | 0.9 |
| **TMT A test (time)** | 3 | 0.59 | 0.01 |
| **TMT B test (score)** | 0.92 | 0.99 | 0.95 |
| **TMT B test (time)** | 4 | 0.88 | 0.02 |

This significant difference in the time taken to perform the TMT A and TMT B tasks was interpreted as a significant slowdown in the speed of information processing in all patients.

#### 5.2.5. Visual-spatial disorders

Compared with control subjects, there was no evidence of a significant deficit in visuo-spatial abilities tested by the REY figure or clock test.

### 5.3. Correlation of CT with other parameters

#### 5.3.1. Correlation of CT with epidemiological factors

A significant correlation was revealed between the different cognitive scores of the affected domains (attention, verbal and visual memory) and the age of the patients (the older the epilepsy patients, the more the scores collapsed ) with a p of 0.01, 0.001 and 0.002 for the 3 domains respectively. Sex was not a factor influencing the degree of impairment, whereas educational level played a significant role and we found that educated subjects had better cognitive scores than illiterate ones ($p<0.05$ for all scores, even intact domains) .

#### 5.3.2. Correlation of CTs with clinical features of the disease

We divided our patients into two groups according to the secondary generalisation of the seizure: ET with secondary generalisation and without secondary generalisation (24 vs 6). At the end of the neuropsychological assessment, we found no significant difference between the two groups, nor between those with mesiotemporal versus lateral temporal seizures.

On the other hand, we found a significant difference in IR and DR scores determined by the 16-word test and the SRT test and the age of onset of ET (ADD) (the earlier the age of onset of seizures, the greater the loss of encoding, storage and retrieval capacity). We also noted a slowdown in VTI in our patients, as well as a worsening of attentional problems and verbal and visual memory as a function of the frequency of attacks per day. The duration of the disease had an impact on the degree of impairment in the various cognitive domains (Table VIII).

Table VIII: Correlations of CT with clinical features of ET

| **Neuropsychological disorders** | ADD | FC | FROM |
|---|---|---|---|
| VTI | **0.005** | **0. 01** | 0.065 |
| ***Verbal* episodic memory disorders** | **0.046** | **0.005** | **0.002** |
| *RL/RI* | | | |
| *SRT* | | | |
| **Episodic memory disorders Visual** | | | |
| *BVMT-R* | **0.02** | **0.005** | **0.009** |
| **Working memory disorders** | | | |
| *Inverse span* | **0.01** | **0.02** | **0.015** |
| **Attention disorders** | | | |
| *Bell* | 0,059 | 0,2 | **0.007** |
| ***Fluency disorders*** | | | |
| *Semantic fluency* | **0.04** | 0.05 | 0.9 |
| *Literal fluency* | 0.8 | 0.7 | 0.64 |

### 5.3.3. Correlation of CT with treatment

We found a significant correlation between Clonazepam intake and scores on different cognitive tests (verbal and visual memory, attention and verbal fluency) (p=0.000, 0.01 and 0.015 respectively). No correlation was observed between the number of treatments (notion of polytherapy) and the scores of different cognitive tests.

5.3.4. Correlation of CT with EEG aspects

We did not find a significant correlation between the presence of electrical abnormalities and the degree of decline in cognitive scores on the various tests.

5.3.5. Correlation of CT with aspects of cerebral MRI

The presence of a temporal lesion on brain MRI was a significant risk factor for the development of CT (p=0.000). Hippocampal sclerosis was the lesion most likely to cause CT, significantly more so than vascular lesions, tumours or other types of hippocampal malformation (p=0.001).

We found that patients with lesions on the left had lower verbal memory scores, slower VTI and lower verbal fluency than those with lesions on the right. Only visual memory was more impaired in the 2nd group. The differences were significant with a p<0.05

Table: correlations between CT and radiological aspects

| **Neuropsychological disorders** | Left lesion group | Group with lesion on the right | p |
|---|---|---|---|
| VTI (TMT A) | 1 min | 3 min | **0.01** |
| **Verbal episodic memory disorders (16-word test)** | | | |
| RI/16 | 4 | 11 | **0.002** |
| RT /48 | 30 | 23.7 | **0.04** |
| RD /16 | 2.1 | 7.56 | **0.02** |
| **Visual episodic memory disorders (BVMT-R test)** | | | |
| RT/ 36 | 26.5 | 18.6 | **0.04** |
| RD/12 | 8.1 | 3.9 | **0.01** |

| | | | |
|---|---|---|---|
| ***Fluency disorders*** | | | |
| *Semantic fluency* | 9.6 | 20.7 | **0.009** |
| *Literal fluency* | 5.2 | 10.6 | **0.04** |

In summary, gender did not interfere with cognitive impairment, but the level of education (NE) had a significant protective effect on cognitive impairment in our group of patients. We observed a worsening of the impairment of the affected domains in our patients compared with the control group, especially according to age, age of onset of epilepsy, seizure frequency, Clonazepam intake and the presence of a lesion on cerebral MRI. Patients with symptomatic left-sided epilepsy had lower scores in most tests, but especially in verbal memory. On the other hand, in patients with lesions on the right, only visual episodic memory was more affected. We did not observe any difference in impairment according to the number of treatments taken or according to the presence of electrical abnormalities on ET.

# DISCUSSION

## DISCUSSION

### 1. Type of cognitive impairment

CT during ET is common. It is currently accepted that one in two patients with ET will develop CTs during their lifetime. On reviewing the literature, we found little research to support or refute the hypothesis of an altered cognitive network using neuro-psychological tests during ET. The majority of these articles either report series with a small number of patients or focus on the study of a single cognitive domain, which in the majority of studies is episodic memory. To date, our work represents the first Tunisian study to investigate CT in ET and the clinico-electro-radiological correlations. A neuropsychological assessment is one of the main investigations in the management of patients with ET. Detection of CT involves a series of tests which, among other things, should explore VTI, attention, short-term and working memory, episodic memory, semantic memory, language fluency, and visuospatial and executive functions. The cognitive assessment methods used differ from one study to another. Several batteries of neuropsychological tests have been used for this assessment, and work has been published to validate the tests [2].

The profile of cognitive impairment found in patients with ET is fairly similar from one patient to another. Several areas are affected. The first area to be affected, in terms of frequency, is episodic memory [3], followed by semantic memory. This is due to the major role played by the hippocampus in all aspects of memory: episodic, spatial and semantic memory [4]. The granular cells in the inner branch of the hippocampus control 78% of a patient's total memory capacity [5]. This latter structure is also involved in cognitive networks that interact dynamically in the ET with functional circuits, including the anterior and lateral part of the temporal lobe, insula, thalamus, cingulate gyrus and prefrontal cortex, resulting in impairment primarily of memory and then of other cognitive domains [3].

By reviewing this long-term memory impairment in detail, the authors found a decline in the three main stages: a disorder of initial learning (encoding), storage (or consolidation) and retrieval (or recollection). This cognitive profile is similar to the hippocampal profile characteristic of Alzheimer's disease (AD). Several authors have reinforced this clinical finding by measuring CSF biomarker levels and studying functional imaging changes in epileptics with an amnestic syndrome. These studies found pathological changes in these epileptics compatible with AD. They concluded that this persistent and progressive cognitive deterioration in some patients followed for ET may be due to an underlying degenerative disease [6]. Some genetic studies have confirmed the similarity between ET with memory impairment and AD. They have reported that verbal and visual episodic memory disorders in patients with drug-resistant ET are linked to the presence of the APOE 4 genotype [7].

In our series we found the same hippocampal profile in 78% of patients.

Semantic memory is a cognitive domain also affected in ET, according to some authors. According to several studies, memory for relative knowledge of famous people is more affected than autobiographical memory. Impairment of this type of memory is due to temporal damage to the neocortex [8]. In our study, we were unable to assess these 2 types of semantic memory due to the lack of validated tests in Arabic and well-established standards. We only have tests that explore semantic matching. In previous studies, we did not specify a list of famous people well known to our Tunisian population.

The slowing of **VTI** is frequently observed in patients with ET. This speed is an aspecific process considered to be an integral part of the other cognitive processes [9]. It is influenced by any cognitive impairment (attention and memory in our study).

Then there is the decline in **attentional capacity**, bearing in mind that attention is a complex neuropsychological process in which several cortical and subcortical networks are involved . Consequently, these attentional functions may be affected in several types of drug-resistant focal epilepsy. Pharmacotherapy, especially polytherapy, decreases attentional performance [10].

**Verbal fluency** is also frequently impaired due to damage to the left anterior temporal lobe, as well as frontotemporal linguistic circuits in the left hemisphere [11].

In our study, we found in our epileptic patients an impairment of VTI, attention and literal fluency, which is in line with previous findings reported in the literature.

Decline in **working memory** capacity is more common in frontal epilepsy. It occurs late in the course of the disease in cases of ET, and is generally absent during the first few years of the disease [10]. In our study, it was least affected in only 53% of cases.

**The executive functions** involved in the control and planning of goal-directed actions were normal in our patients because they are controlled essentially by the frontal lobes. The deterioration of these functions in ET reported by some authors may be explained by diffusion from the temporal EZ to the frontal cortex. Other authors have linked the presence of executive function deficits to atrophy or metabolic changes in the prefrontal cortex or in the circuit linking the hippocampus to the thalamus encountered during ET [12].

Visual-constructive disorders were not frequently studied. Few studies have reported a decline in these functions. In our study, we tested these functions so that we could study most cognitive domains and, above all, so that we had a validated test with precise norms. We did not observe any visuo-constructive disorders in our epileptic patients [13].

2. Clinical correlations

The complexity of the multiple factors and their interactions makes it impossible to target a single etiology of cognitive impairment in patients with this type of epilepsy. Among the best-studied variables likely to play a role in this decline in cognitive ability are the patient's age, the age of onset of the epilepsy, the duration of the course of the disease, the frequency of seizures, antiepileptic drugs and the response to these treatments, and the presence of a lesion, particularly a mesiotemporal lesion and its laterality.

### 2.1. Correlations between CT and epidemiological factors

#### 2.1.1. Age :

Memory complaints were correlated with age. Multivariate analysis confirmed that cognitive decline was more severe in older patients [14]. Some authors explain this correlation by a physiopathological mechanism similar to that of AD, based on studies of animal models and anatomopathology of surgical parts. These studies have shown an accumulation of amyloid plaques and an increase in Tau and phosphorylated Tau proteins, which is greater in older epileptics.

The age of onset of the disease was also an aggravating factor in CT, the earlier the onset of epilepsy, the more severe the degree of involvement [15].

In our work, we found a correlation between cognitive decline, patient age and the age of onset of the disease. These results are in line with those reported in the literature [16].

#### 2.1.2. Gender

Studies comparing the degree of cognitive impairment according to sex have not revealed significant correlations [17]. Our study is in the same vein and found no difference in the degree of cognitive impairment between the 2 sexes.

#### 2.1.3. Educational level

Several studies around the world suggest that the most highly educated subjects have a lower risk of developing CD. In fact, cognitive reserves increase with the level of education, enabling the subject to use, for example, more strategies in recognition functions [18]. In our study, we found that subjects with a secondary education or higher had better cognitive scores than those with a primary education.

### 2.2.Correlation of CT with clinical features of the disease

2.2.1. CT correlations with the diffusion of the EZ

Some studies have shown that cognitive performance is poorer in patients with focal seizures with secondary generalisation [19].

In our study, the majority of our patients had generalised diffusion and we did not find this significant correlation between the diffusion of the EZ and the severity of CT in the different areas.

2.2.2. Correlations between CT and the duration of the epileptic course

Studies also show that there is a correlation between the duration of the disease and cognitive impairment. Several authors have found that the degree of neuropsychological decline was significantly correlated with the duration of the disease [20]. which was the case for our patients, the study by jokeit and Ebner, in which the authors included 209 patients divided into 2 groups (epilepsy with more or less than 30 years of progression) [21] and the study by aikia et al of 2 groups, one of 39 newly diagnosed untreated epileptics and the other of 16 epileptics followed over a period of more than 10 years [22]. Some post-mortem anatomopathological studies have supported this hypothesis, showing that there is neuronal loss in layers II and III of the entorhinal cortex over time and during the course of the epilepsy [23].

2.2.3. Correlations between CT and seizure frequency

Data on the impact of CEs on the intellectual faculties of patients with ET remain controversial, depending on the series. Several studies were unable to show a correlation between seizure frequency and CT. In contrast, other studies have shown an association between seizure frequency, memory impairment and attentional difficulties. These findings were also found in our sample. The relationship between hippocampal damage during ET and seizure frequency goes in both directions. Firstly, this high frequency of seizures potentiates the effects of mesiotemporal damage on the decline of episodic memory without affecting semantic memory (knowledge of famous people) or attention or executive functions [24].

The reverse is also true. The majority of studies on animal models have suggested that the noradrenergic nervous system has an anticonvulsant effect and that the hippocampus is the only structure that receives these noradrenergic innervations from the locus coeruleus. The loss of hippocampal neurons in ET can lead to impaired noradrenergic function, which has a convulsant effect by increasing the frequency of ECs [6].

### 2.3 Correlation of CT with treatment

The long-term effects of anti-epileptic drugs on cognition are widely debated. Some studies have shown that these cognitive disorders are only related to the use of antiepileptic drugs. Others have refuted this hypothesis, showing that even in patients not taking antiepileptic drugs, these cognitive disorders exist. The risk of adverse cognitive effects is more severe in patients taking multiple medications. The dosage and serum level of treatments also have a negative impact on cognitive capacity, especially attentional capacity [25]. Several studies have compared the effect of different antiepileptic drugs on cognition. Benzodiazepines and barbiturates have been shown to be safe in terms of cognitive slowing [26]. In the study by Meador et al, the authors showed that phenytoin, carbamazepine and sodium valporate were less harmful than the latter. Uncontrolled studies show that there is no difference between the effects of phenytoin and carbamazepine on cognition [27].

The new generations of anti-epileptic drugs are likely to have a greater benefit on cognitive ability than the first generation, but these data are patchy and based on small series [28]. Certain side effects may be caused even by this family of drugs, such as somnolence with gabapentin, and slowing, memory and language problems with topiramate. Gabapentin and lamotrigine had less cognitive impact than topiramate [29].

In our study, we found low cognitive scores in all domains in epileptic patients taking clonazepam without any effect of the number of treatments received.

## 3. Correlation of CTs with aspects of EEG :

Studies have found a correlation between cognitive decline and the presence of inter-critical electrical discharges (EDs). These spikes and spike waves may be continuous in favour of sub-clinical seizures that interfere with specific functional hippocampal word retrieval networks by impairing these faculties.

These discharges can also cause an acute effect in the form of transient cognitive impairment. Its chronic repercussions remain a subject of debate, with some studies showing a decline in global functions (deterioration in IQ) [30], while others have studied the correlations between these EDs according to their topography and the cognitive domain studied: only impairment of phonemic and semantic fluency was correlated with the presence of EDs in the left anterior temporal cortex [31]. More recently, Kleen et al. have reported that hippocampal intercritical ED can disrupt storage and retrieval, but not encoding [32]. Mameniskiene et al demonstrated that the presence of temporal EDs can accelerate the forgetting of word lists and complex patterns such as Rey's pattern [33]. Several molecular biology studies have sought to explain these correlations. These have concluded that the sodium channel cleaving enzyme causing ET and the amyloid precursor protein (APP) cleaving enzyme will activate the processing of APP to produce amyloid Aβ peptides. This cleavage is associated with aberrant EEG activity and cognitive deficits.

In the normal state, Aβ is regulated presynaptically. However, a higher concentration of Aβ worked in the opposite direction and caused synaptic depression leading to network instability and promoting synchrony, which predispose to epileptiform activity **[34]**.

**↑enzyme de clivage**
**des canaux de sodium**
**protéine précurseur de l'amyloïde (APP) → Aβ amyloïde → ↑ activité épileptiforme**

Other authors disagree and reject the impact of intercritical EDs on long-term memory **[35]**. In our series, we did not reveal any inter-critical discharges. Only slow waves and diffuse slowing, which were not correlated with cognitive deterioration.

4. Correlation of CT with aspects of brain MRI

Much of the cognitive impairment that occurs in people with ET is related to its underlying aetiology (tumours, vascular malformations, arachnoid cysts, dysplasia and hippocampal atrophy measured by volumetric study) **[12]**.

A significant correlation has been reported in the literature between the presence of a lesion on MRI, especially hippocampal sclerosis, and the degree of cognitive decline **[36]**. Not only is the presence of HS a predictive factor for CT, but the extent of decline is related to the degree of neuronal loss in the hippocampus and adjacent temporal structures (memory is strongly affected if the loss of granular cells in the hippocampus exceeds 60%) **[37]**. This can be reinforced by the results of functional and PET-FDG imaging, as well as the degree of hippocampal atrophy calculated by volumetric measurements.

In our study, we also found that the presence of symptomatic epilepsy is a predisposing factor for the onset of CT. In our study, as in the literature, HS was the most harmful lesion for cognitive functions.

It is not easy to show a link between damage to a given neuropsychological area and damage to a specific anatomical structure in the brain.

Several authors have compared the cognitive profile of patients with a left ET with those with a right ET. Firstly, overall cognitive decline is greater if the EZ is located in the dominant hemisphere **[38]**. In addition, studies have shown that in right-handed patients, it is classically recognised that the memory deficit predominates on verbal material in the case of a left lateralized EZ, whereas the visual memory impairment is more severe if the EZ is on the right **[39]**. In our sample, we reported similar findings.

5. Impact of CT on surgical management

Changes in memory after temporal lobe surgery were determined mainly by analysing the results of cognitive tests. A significant improvement in post-operative memory indices (after hippocampectomy) was observed in 23.3-36.6% of patients and the improvement in memory was equivalent between the right and left epileptogenic zone groups and between verbal and visual abilities **[40]**.

# CONCLUSION

## CONCLUSION

ET is a serious neurological condition with long-term implications for health and well-being. It is a cause of disability in young people, not only because of the drug-resistant seizures associated with the difficult-to-control disease, but also because of the CT that affects patients' social and professional activities. In fact, almost half of all people with epilepsy suffer from these disorders. They preferentially affect all aspects of memory. In our study, based on clinical data (history, neuropsychological evaluation), we found cognitive impairment in the majority of patients by comparing their performance with that of a matched control group (age, sex and educational level). The impairment was mainly in VTI, memory, verbal fluency and attention. Cognitive domains controlled by the anterior and posterior cortices, especially executive and visuo-spatial functions, were intact. These CTs were generally more severe in older patients and those with an earlier age of onset of epilepsy. The level of education had a significant protective effect in our group of patients. Gender did not interfere with cognitive impairment. We observed a worsening of the cognitive domains affected, especially as a function of the frequency of seizures and the duration of the epilepsy. We did not observe any difference in impairment between the 2 groups (with or without secondary generalisation). The presence of a slowdown in background EEG activity was not significantly correlated with the degree of cognitive decline in the various domains. The number of background treatments (polytherapy) had no effect on the cognitive complaints of our patients, but the prescription of benzodiazepines was the most harmful. These clinical factors had an impact on the degree of impairment, and the data provided by magnetic resonance imaging (MRI) also had a decisive role to play in determining the nature of these cognitive disorders.

We found a correlation between the presence of a temporal lesion on brain MRI and the degree of cognitive decline, especially in verbal episodic memory. Hippocampal sclerosis was the lesion most likely to cause these CTs. There was also a correlation between the nature of the area affected and the laterality of the epileptogenic zone. Patients in whom the EZ was located on the left had lower scores in most tests, especially verbal memory tests, whereas those with an EZ on the right were more likely to have visual episodic memory impairment. These findings enabled us to demonstrate the presence of neuropsychological mapping within the different brain regions. If ET appears at an early age, it can activate processes for reorganising the cognitive map with some effectiveness.

A number of future analyses could complement our study in order to better specify the differences between children and adults and better understand this reorganisation. We plan to complete the postoperative exploration in order to better highlight the effect of surgery on cognitive functions.

A correlation study between these CTs and functional imaging abnormalities (PET-SCANN) is also desirable.

In our study, we looked at correlations between the degree of impairment and treatment. Further investigation after a change in treatment may confirm the harmful effect of certain anti-epileptic drugs on cognitive abilities. The aim is to control the epileptic component of the disease, but also to preserve cognitive function. Cognitive management must be comprehensive and involve several levels. There is no consensual neuropsychological re-education programme, but there are many possible approaches: group or individual, computerised or ecological, etc.

The therapeutic approach must involve medical, psychological and social care, which is essential, especially at an early age, to activate compensatory mechanisms and overcome functional deficiencies in certain networks, bearing in mind that training in a specific cognitive area can improve cognitive skills in several other areas.

# REFERENCES

1. THOMPSON PJ, CORCORAN R. EVERYDAY MEMORY FAILURES IN PEOPLE WITH EPILEPSY. EPILEPSIA. 1992;33:18-20.
2. Zita Bouman et al. Clinical utility of the Wechsler Memory Scale- Fourth Edition (WMS-IV) in patients with intraclable temporal lobe epilepsy. Epilepsy and Behavior. 2016; 55: 178-182
3. Tanja S. Kellermann et al. Mapping the neuropsychological profile of temporal lobe epilepsy using cognitive network topology and graph theory. Epilepsy & Behavior. 2016; 63: 9-16
4. Squire LR, Stark CE, Clark RE. The medial temporal lobe. Annu Rev Neurosci. 2004; 27:279-306.
5. Pauli E, Hildebrandt M, Romstock J, Stefan H, Blumcke I. Deficient memory acquisition in temporal lobe epilepsy is predicted by hippocampal granule cell loss. Neurology. 2006; 67:1383-1389.
6. Bin-Yin Li, and Sheng-Di Chen. Potential Similarities in Temporal Lobe Epilepsy and Alzheimer's Disease: From Clinic to Pathology. American Journal of Alzheimer's Disease & Other Dementias. 2015 : 1-6
7. Bungenberg J et al. Gene expression variance in hippocampal tissue of temporal lobe epilepsy patients corresponds to differential memory performance. Neurobiol Dis. 2016; 86:121-30.
8. Anna Rita Giovagnoli, Alessandra Erbetta, Flavio Villani, Giuliano Avanzini. Semantic memory in partial epilepsy: verbal and non-verbal Deficits and neuroanatomical relationships. 2005; 43: 1482-1492
9. Cassel A1, Morris R2, Koutroumanidis M3, Kopelman M ; Forgetting in temporal lobe epilepsy: When does it become accelerated? Cortex. 2016;78:70-84

10. S. Lippé, M. Lasson. Assessment of drug-resistant partial epilepsy: neuropsychological investigations. Rev neurol. 2004; 160:144-153

11. Besson P, Dinkelacker V, Valabregue R, Thivard L, Leclerc X, Baulac M, et al. Structural connectivity differences in left and right temporal lobe epilepsy. Neuroimage. 2014 ; 100:135-44.

12. Dinkelacker V, Xin X, Baulac M, Samson S, Dupont S. Interictal epileptic discharge correlates with global and frontal cognitive dysfunction in temporal lobe epilepsy. Epilepsy Behav. 2016; 62:197-203

13. Zhao F, Kang H, You L, Rastogi P, Venkatesh DChandra M. Neuropsychological deficits in temporal lobe epilepsy: A comprehensive review. Ann Indian Acad Neurol. 2014;17:374-82.

14. L. Valton and C-R Mascott. What is the role of neuropsychological assessment in the management of patients with drug-resistant partial epilepsy? Rev Neurol. 2004; 160: 154-63

15. Lespinet V, Bresson C, N'Kaoua B, Rougier A, Claverie B. Effect of age of onset of temporal lobe epilepsy on the severity and the nature of preoperative memory deficits. Neuropsychologia. 2002;40: 1591-600.

16. Coras R, Blümcke I. Clinicopathological subtypes of hippocampal sclerosis in temporal lobe epilepsy and their differential impact on memory impairment. Neuroscience. 2015;309:153-61

17. Bergin PS1, Thompson PJ, Baxendale SA, Fish DR, Shorvon SD. Remote memory in epilepsy. Epilepsia. 2000;41:231-9.

18. Loiseau P, Signoret JL, Strube E, Broustet D, Dartigues JF. New approaches to the study of memory impairment in epileptics. Rev Neurol ; 1982; 138:387-400.

19. Bergin P et al. Remote memory in epilepsy. Epilepsia, 41: 231-239

20. Helmstaedter C, Elger CE. Chronic temporal lobe epilepsy: a neurodevelopmental or progressively dementing disease? Brain . 2009;132: 2822-30.
21. Jokeit H, Ebner A. Long term effects of refractory temporal lobe epilepsy on cognitive abilities: a cross sectional study. J Neurol Neurosurg Psychiatry. 1999 Jul;67:44-50.
22. Aikiä M, Salmenperä T, Partanen K, Kälviäinen R. Verbal Memory in Newly Diagnosed Patients and Patients with Chronic Left Temporal Lobe Epilepsy. Epilepsy Behav. 2001 Feb;2 :20-27.
23. LiBY, Chen SD. Potential Similarities in Temporal Lobe Epilepsy and Alzheimer's Disease: From Clinic to Pathology. Am J Alzheimers Dis Other Demen. 2015;30 :723-8.
24. Voltzenlogel V, Vignal JP, Hirsch E. Manning The influence of seizure frequency on anterograde and remote memory in mesial temporal lobe epilepsy. Seizure. 2014; 23: 792-8.
25. Hermann B1, Meador KJ, Gaillard WD, Cramer JA. Cognition across the lifespan: antiepileptic drugs, epilepsy, or both? Epilepsy Behav. 2010;17:1-5.
26. Loring DW1, Marino SE, Drane DL, Parfitt D, Finney GR, Meador KJ. Lorazepam effects on Word Memory Test performance: a randomized, double-blind, placebo-controlled, crossover trial. Clin Neuropsychol. 2011 Jul;25(5):799-811.

27. Meador KJ. Comparative cognitive effects of carbamazepine and phenytoin in healthy adults. Neurology. 1991;41:1537-40.
28. Helmstaedter C, Witt JA. Cognitive outcome of antiepileptic treatment with levetiracetam versus carbamazepine monotherapy: a non-interventional surveillance trial. Epilepsy Behav. 2010 May;18(1-2):74-80.

29. Brunbech L1, Sabers A. Effect of antiepileptic drugs on cognitive function in individuals with epilepsy: a comparative review of newer versus older agents. Drugs. 2002;62:593-604.

30. Dinkelacker V, Dupont S, Samson S. The new approach to classification of focal epilepsies: Epileptic discharge and disconnectivity in relation to cognition. Epilepsy Behav. 2016; 5050(16)30435-8

31. 1, Arends J. Effects of epileptiform EEG discharges on cognitive function: is the concept of "transient cognitive impairment" still valid? Epilepsy Behav. 2004; 1:25-34.

32. Kleen JK, Hippocampal interictal epileptiform activity disrupts cognition in humans. Neurology. 2013 Jul 2;81(1):18-24

33. Mameniskiene R, Jatuzis D, Kaubrys G, Budrys V. The decay of memory between delayed and long-term recall in patients with temporal lobe epilepsy. Epilepsy Behav. 2006;8:278-88.

34. Bin-Yin Li1, and Sheng-Di Chen. Potential Similarities in Temporal Lobe Epilepsy and Alzheimer's Disease: From Clinic to Pathology. American Journal of Alzheimer's Disease & Other Dementias; 30(8):723-8.

35. Provinciali L, Signorino M, Censori B, Ceravolo G, Del Pesce M. Recognition impairment correlated with short bisynchronous epileptic discharges. Epilepsia. 1991; 32(5):684-9.

36. C. Helmstaedter and C. E. Elger. Chronic temporal lobe epilepsy: a neurodevelopmental or progressively dementing disease? Brain. 2009;132:2822-30.

37. Coras R1, Blümcke I. Clinico-pathological subtypes of hippocampal sclerosis in temporal lobe epilepsy and their differential impact on memory impairment. Neuroscience. 2015; 309:153-61

38. Mameniškienė R, Rimšienė J, Puronaitė R Cognitive changes in people with temporal lobe epilepsy over a 13-year period. Epilepsy Behav. 2016;63:89-97.
39. Kellermann TS et al. Mapping the neuropsychological profile of temporal lobe epilepsy using cognitive network topology andgraph theory. Epilepsy Behav. 2016 Oct;63:9-16.
40. Khalil AF, Iwasaki M, Nishio Y, Jin K, Nakasato NTominaga T. Verbal Dominant Memory Impairment and Low Risk for Post-Operative Memory Worsening in Both Left and Right Temporal Lobe Epilepsy Associated with Hippocampal Sclerosis. Neurol Med Chir 2016 15; 56(11):716-723

# SUMMARY

**Issue:** Temporal epilepsy (TE) is a disabling disease, characterised above all by its drug resistance. Cognitive impairment (CI) affects around half of patients and has an impact on their daily lives, constituting an invisible handicap. Neuropsychological tests are used to identify cognitive impairment. Several socio-epidemiological, clinical, electrical and radiological factors interfere with the onset of cognitive decline.

**Aim:** The aim of our work is to evaluate the presence, extent and type of CTs in ET patients and then to study their possible correlations with epidemioclinical data on the one hand and imaging data on the other.

**Methods:** We conducted a cross-sectional study over a 6-month period (May-November 2022), including patients followed at the Neurology Department of the Habib Bourguiba University Hospital in Sfax for ET according to the criteria of the International League Against Epilepsy (ILAE). Our patients underwent a careful clinical examination and a thorough neuropsychological evaluation. All patients had an EEG and brain MRI.

**Results:** We enrolled 32 patients (13 men and 19 women). The average age of our patients was 35 years [19-92 years]. Compared with the neuropsychological scores obtained in the control group, we found marked cognitive impairment in our patients, particularly in the areas of VTI, attention and, above all, verbal and visual episodic memory. Executive capacity and visuo-spatial perception were intact. We related the severity of this impairment to a number of socio-epidemiological factors (age, age of onset of ET and educational level) and to the severity of the epilepsy (seizure frequency and drug resistance). We found significant correlations between Clonazepan use and the degree of cognitive impairment, especially attentional impairment. The presence of a temporal lesion, especially hippocampal sclerosis, was the most common cause of episodic memory impairment. The laterality of the epileptogenic zone characterised the nature of the episodic memory affected: if this EZ is located on the left, the impairment is mainly verbal, whereas if it is on the right, we noted a visual memory complaint, given that the left lesion is more harmful.

**Conclusion:** At the end of our work, we emphasise the importance of identifying CT in order to improve subsequent management and minimise its impact on a population that is often young and active.

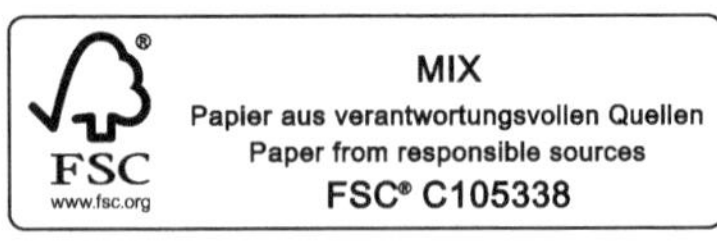


Printed by Books on Demand GmbH, Norderstedt / Germany